GOUT COOKBOOK

MAIN COURSE – 80 + Low Purine Breakfast, Main Course, Dessert and Snacks Recipes

TABLE OF CONTENTS

Introduction

Gout recipes for personal enjoyment but also for family enjoyment. You will love them for sure for how easy it is to prepare them.

ROASTED CHERRY & RICOTTA TARTINE

Serves: **2**

Prep Time: **20**   Minutes

Cook Time: **30**   Minutes

Total Time: **50**   Minutes

INGREDIENTS

- ~ 2 cups cherries
- ~ 1 tablespoon honey
- ~ 1 tsp lemon zest
- ~ 1 tablespoon lemon juice
- ~ 1 tsp olive oil
- ~ salt
- ~ 4 slices bread
- ~ 1 cup part-skim ricotta cheese
- ~ 1 tsp thyme
- ~ ½ cup almonds

DIRECTIONS

1. **Preheat the oven to 375 F**

2. In a bowl toss with lemon juice, oil, honey and roast them for about 12-15 minutes
3. Toast bread and top with lemon zest, ricotta cheese, cherries, thyme, almonds, and salt
4. Drizzle with honey and serve

MORNING MANGO BOWL

Serves:	*4*	
Prep Time:	*10*	Minutes
Cook Time:	*10*	Minutes
Total Time:	*20*	Minutes

INGREDIENTS

- ½ cup mango
- ¼ cup Greek Yogurt
- ½ cup banana
- ½ cup unsweetened almond milk
- 4 tablespoons almonds
- ½ tsp allspice

- ½ cup raspberries
- ¼ tsp honey

DIRECTIONS

1. In a blender add all ingredients and blend until smooth
2. Pour the mango yogurt into a bowl and serve with raspberries and almonds

BROWNIE COOKIES

Serves: **4**

Prep Time: **10** Minutes

Cook Time: **30** Minutes

Total Time: **40** Minutes

INGREDIENTS

- 2 oz. unsweetened chocolate
- 1 stick butter
- 1 cup Splenda

- 1 egg
- ¼ tsp vanilla
- ¾ cup whole-wheat flour
- ½ tsp baking soda
- ¼ cup chocolate chips
- ¼ cup walnuts

DIRECTIONS

1. Preheat the oven to 325 F
2. Microwave chocolate for 30 seconds
3. In another bowl mix Splenda, butter, vanilla, and the egg
4. Stir in melted chocolate, baking soda, flour, chocolate chips, and nuts
5. Drop teaspoons of batter onto the baking sheet and bake for 10-12 minutes
6. Remove and serve

Serves:	*8*
Prep Time:	*10* Minutes
Cook Time:	*20* Minutes
Total Time:	*30* Minutes

INGREDIENTS

- 1 cup oats
- 1 cup flour
- 1 tsp baking powder
- ½ tsp salt
- ¾ cup brown sugar
- 1 egg
- 1 cup skim milk
- 1/2 cup vegetable oil
- 1 carrot
- 1 cup raisins
- ¼ cup walnuts

DIRECTIONS

1. **Preheat the oven to 375 F**

2. In a bowl mix flour, oats, salt, baking powder, and sugar
3. In another bowl beat eggs and carrots, vegetable oil and milk
4. Stir wet ingredients into dry ingredients and mix well
5. Stir in walnuts raisins and divide batter into 8-10 muffin cups
6. Bake for 18-20 minutes, remove and serve

CONFETTI WARPS

Serves: *4*

Prep Time: *10* Minutes

Cook Time: *30* Minutes

Total Time: *40* Minutes

INGREDIENTS

- 1 oz. ham
- 1 oz. turkey
- 1 oz. Swiss cheese
- 1 egg

- 3 leaves romaine lettuce
- ½ cup yellow bell pepper
- ½ cup red onion
- ½ cup cucumber
- 1 tomato
- 1 carrot
- 1 tablespoon salad dressing
- 2 large tomato wraps

DIRECTIONS

1. Roll ham, turkey and Swiss cheese and cut into thin strips, toss with vegetables and roll your tortilla
2. Place a tablespoon of dressing on your tortilla

Serves: **4**

Prep Time: **10**   Minutes

Cook Time: **30**   Minutes

Total Time: **40**   Minutes

INGREDIENTS

- 1 egg
- ¼ cup yogurt
- ¼ cup brown sugar
- 1 cup quick oats
- 1 tablespoon flaxseed
- ½ cup chocolate chips

DIRECTIONS

1. In a bowl whisk yogurt, egg, and sugar
2. In a blender add oats, flaxseed, chocolate chips, egg mixture and blend until smooth
3. Spread mixture in a pan and bake at 325 F for 25 min
4. Remove, cut into bars and serve

Serves: **4**

Prep Time: **10** Minutes

Cook Time: **30** Minutes

Total Time: **40** Minutes

INGREDIENTS

- 2 cups water
- 1 cup brown rice
- 1 cup milk
- 1 cup Splenda
- 1 cup crystallized ginger

DIRECTIONS

1. In a saucepan bring water and rice to a boil, reduce heat and cook for 25-30 minutes
2. Stir in Splenda while rice is cooking
3. Add milk, ginger and spend and cook until milk is absorbed
4. Remove from heat garnish with orange slices and serve

Serves: **3**

Prep Time: **10** Minutes

Cook Time: **35** Minutes

Total Time: **45** Minutes

INGREDIENTS

- 2 egg whites
- ½ cup Splenda
- ½ tsp vanilla
- 1 tablespoon lemon curd

DIRECTIONS

1. In a bowl beat egg whites, add Splenda and continue to mix
2. Stir in vanilla and mix well
3. Drop mixture using a pipe onto a baking sheet making around 10-12 portions
4. Bake at 275 F for 25-30 minutes
5. Remove and serve

Serves: *2*

Prep Time: *10*   Minutes

Cook Time: *10*   Minutes

Total Time: *20*   Minutes

INGREDIENTS

- 1 lemon
- 1 packet sweet
- 1 cup water
- 1 cup ice cubes

DIRECTIONS

1. Cut lemon in half and squeeze the juice into a glass
2. Add sweetener, water, and ice cubes
3. Mix well, garnish with a strawberry and serve

Serves: *8*

Prep Time: *10*   Minutes

Cook Time: *35*   Minutes

Total Time: *45*   Minutes

INGREDIENTS

- 1 15 oz. can pumpkin
- ½ cup egg substitute
- ¾ cup sugar
- 1 tsp cinnamon
- ¼ tsp ground ginger
- ½ tsp nutmeg
- ½ tsp cloves
- 1 12 oz. can evaporated skim milk

CRUST

- 1 cup flour
- 2 tablespoons water
- ½ cup shortening

DIRECTIONS

1. **Preheat the oven to 400 F**

2.   Place shortening, water, and flour into a bowl and mix well and form a ball

3.   Let it stand for 20-30 minutes and then roll crust in a pan

4.   In a whisk together pumpkin, sugar, egg substitute, evaporated milk and mix well

5.   Pour mixture into pie shell and bake for 35 minutes

6.   Remove and serve

FRUIT TARTS

Serves: *2*

Prep Time: *10*   Minutes

Cook Time: *20*   Minutes

Total Time: *30*   Minutes

INGREDIENTS

- 1 tart apple
- 1 tablespoon Splenda
- ½ tsp cinnamon
- 10 wonton wrappers

DIRECTIONS

1. Preheat the oven to 325 F
2. Grate the apples and sprinkle with cinnamon and Splenda
3. Fill a muffin pan with grated apple and bake for 10-12 minutes, remove and serve

MORNING ICE TEA

Serves: *1*

Prep Time: *10*   Minutes

Cook Time: *10*   Minutes

Total Time: *20*   Minutes

INGREDIENTS

- 3 cups cold water
- 2 peaches tea bags
- 1 cup ice cubes

DIRECTIONS

1. Pour water, ice cubes and tea bags in a glass
2. After 2-3 minutes remove tea bags and serve

KIWI SPRITZER

Serves: **4**

Prep Time: **10** Minutes

Cook Time: **30** Minutes

Total Time: **40** Minutes

INGREDIENTS

- 1 kiwi
- ½ cup strawberries
- ¾ seltzer
- 1 cup ice cubes

DIRECTIONS

1. In a bowl mash kiwi and strawberries
2. Pour juice, ice, and top with seltzer

3. Mix well and serve

FRENCH DRESSING

Serves: **4**

Prep Time: **10**   Minutes

Cook Time: **10**   Minutes

Total Time: **20**   Minutes

INGREDIENTS

-   ½ cup ketchup
-   ½ cup oil
-   ½ cup white vinegar
-   1 tsp lemon juice
-   4 bread slices

DIRECTIONS

1. In a bowl stir all ingredients until well combined
2. Dip the bread into the mixture

3. Fry bread for 1-2 minutes per side

4. Remove and serve

Serves: **4**

Prep Time: **10** Minutes

Cook Time: **30** Minutes

Total Time: **40** Minutes

INGREDIENTS

- 1 cup dark rum
- 1 tsp lemon rind
- ¾ cup artificial sweetener
- 1 cup walnuts
- 1 cup pecans
- 3 cups cranberries

DIRECTIONS

1. In a saucepan add Splenda, rum and bring to a boil
2. Add cranberries, lemon zest and simmer on low heat for 12-15 minutes
3. Add nuts cook for 2-3 minutes, remove and serve

MORNING CRANBERRY SALAD

Serves: **4**

Prep Time: **10** Minutes

Cook Time: **30** Minutes

Total Time: **40** Minutes

INGREDIENTS

- 1 can unsweetened pineapple
- 1 package cherry gelatin
- 1 tablespoon lemon juice
- ½ cup sweetener
- 1 cup cranberries
- 1 orange
- 1 cup celery

- ½ cup pecans

DIRECTIONS

1. **In a bowl mix all salad ingredients**
2. **Serve when ready**

BANANA SPLIT

Serves: **2**

Prep Time: **10** Minutes

Cook Time: **10** Minutes

Total Time: **20** Minutes

INGREDIENTS

- 2 bananas
- 1 cup strawberries
- 1 cup blackberries
- 1 cup chopped pineapple
- 1 cup coconut milk
- 1 tablespoon whole grain granola

-   ¼ ounce roasted coconut chips

DIRECTIONS

1. Slice the bananas and place them into a bowl
2. Divide the strawberries, blackberries, and pineapple and place it in the bottom of the bowl
3. Top with yogurt and divide the granola and coconut chips between the bananas

CHAI-SPICED PEAR OATMEAL

Serves: *2*

Prep Time: *10*   Minutes

Cook Time: *30*   Minutes

Total Time: *40*   Minutes

INGREDIENTS

-   1 cup oats
-   ½ tsp ground cinnamon
-   1 tsp maple syrup
-   1 tablespoon walnut halves
-   2 tsp coconut oil

- 1 Anjou pear spiralized
- 1 cup almond milk
- ½ tsp vanilla extract

DIRECTIONS

1. In a saucepan boil water and add oats for another 10 minutes
2. In a skillet heat coconut oil over medium heat and add almond milk, pear noodles, cinnamon, maple syrup, and vanilla extract
3. Stir to simmer for about 10-15 minutes
4. In another skillet place walnuts and cook for 5-6 minutes, remove from the pan when ready
5. Place the oatmeal in a bowl and top with pear mixture and toasted walnuts

Serves: **4**

Prep Time: **10** Minutes

Cook Time: **10** Minutes

Total Time: **20** Minutes

INGREDIENTS

- ½ cup rice flour
- 1 tsp baking soda
- 1 banana
- ½ tsp salt
- 2 tablespoons oil
- ½ cup milk
- 1 tsp cider vinegar
- 1 egg
- ½ cup quinoa flakes
- 1 tablespoon honey

DIRECTIONS

1. In a bowl mix all dry ingredients
2. Separate egg yolk from egg white and beat egg whites
3. Mix egg yolk with milk, honey, wet fruit and add dry ingredients to mixture

4. Add cider vinegar and mix gently
5. Pour mixture into waffle iron
6. When ready remove and serve

BREAKFAST BISCUITS

Serves: **12**

Prep Time: **10**   Minutes

Cook Time: **15**   Minutes

Total Time: **25**   Minutes

INGREDIENTS

- 2 cups flour
- 1 tsp xantham gum
- ½ tsp salt
- 4 tablespoons margarine
- 1 tablespoon baking powder
- 1 tsp sugar

DIRECTIONS

1. Preheat oven to 425 F
2. Toss together all ingredients, gather into a ball
3. Form small biscuits and bake for 12-15 minutes
4. Remove and serve

CHICKEN PIZZA

Serves: **2**

Prep Time: **10**   Minutes

Cook Time: **20**   Minutes

Total Time: **30**   Minutes

INGREDIENTS

- 1 ready-made pizza crust
- 1 tsp olive oil
- 1 cup onion
- 14 cup red pepper strips
- 1 cup chicken
- ¼ cup barbecue sauce
- 1 cup mozzarella cheese
- topping of any choice

DIRECTIONS

1. Preheat the oven to 425 F
2. In a frying pan add pepper strips, onion, chicken and cook on low heat

3. Cook until ready and remove from heat
4. Place crust on a cookie sheet and spread barbecue sauce, and the rest of ingredients on the crust
5. Top with mozzarella and bake for 12-15 minutes
6. Remove and serve

CIABATTA PIZZA

Serves: **2**

Prep Time: **10** Minutes

Cook Time: **20** Minutes

Total Time: **30** Minutes

INGREDIENTS

- 1 loaf ciabatta
- 1 cup tomato sauce
- 1 zucchini
- ½ cup mushrooms
- 1 cup mozzarella cheese
- 1 tablespoon basil

DIRECTIONS

1. Preheat the oven to 375 F
2. Cum ciabatta lengthwise and place on a cookie sheet
3. Spread sauce, zucchini, mushrooms on each one and top with mozzarella
4. Sprinkle basil, bake for 12-15 minutes, remove and serve

FIESTA SHRIMP

Serves: *2*
Prep Time: *10*   Minutes

Cook Time: *10*   Minutes

Total Time: *20*   Minutes

INGREDIENTS

- 3 oz. shrimp
- ½ cup zucchini
- ½ cup fiesta garden salsa
- ½ oz. Monterey Jack cheese

- cilantro
- 1 tortilla

DIRECTIONS

1. In a bowl add zucchini, shrimp and salsa
2. Microwave for 4-5 minutes, remove and add grated cheese
3. Sprinkle cilantro and pour mixture over tortilla
4. Serve when ready

GRILLED SALMON STEAKS

Serves: *2*
Prep Time: *10*   Minutes

Cook Time: *10*   Minutes

Total Time: *20*   Minutes

INGREDIENTS

- 2 salmon steaks

- 1 tablespoon dipping sauce
- 1 tsp cooking oil

DIRECTIONS

1. **Preheat grill**
2. **Baste salmon steaks with sauce and cook for 5-6 minutes**
3. **Remove and serve**

ORIENTAL GREENS

Serves: *2*
Prep Time: *10*   Minutes

Cook Time: *10*   Minutes

Total Time: *20*   Minutes

INGREDIENTS

- ½ cup green beans
- ¼ cup snow peas

- 1 cup cauliflower florets
- 1 cup water chestnuts
- 2 radishes
- 2 scallions
- ½ cup red onion
- 1 tsp powdered ginger
- ½ cup rice wine vinegar

DIRECTIONS

1. In a bowl mix cauliflower floret, onions, chestnuts, radish, beans and snow peas
2. In another bowl mix rice wine vinegar, ginger, pour over vegetables and mix well
3. Mix well and serve

Serves: **2**

Prep Time: **10** Minutes

Cook Time: **20** Minutes

Total Time: **30** Minutes

INGREDIENTS

- 13 oz. pizza dough
- 1 tablespoon cornmeal
- ¼ cup ricotta cheese
- 1 lb. shrimp
- 5 cloves garlic
- 1 cup mozzarella cheese
- 1 tablespoon dried basil

DIRECTIONS

1. Preheat the oven to 375 F
2. In a baking pan sprinkle cornmeal and add the pizza dough, bake for 6-8 minutes
3. Remove and cover pizza with mozzarella, ricotta, garlic and sprinkle with basil
4. Bake for 12-15 minutes, remove and serve

Serves: *2*

Prep Time: *10* Minutes

Cook Time: *10* Minutes

Total Time: *20* Minutes

INGREDIENTS

- 1/3 cup vinegar
- ¼ cup whipping cream
- 2 eggs
- ½ cup Splenda
- pinch of salt
- 1 tablespoon butter
- 1 lb. cabbage

DIRECTIONS

1. In a saucepan add vinegar, whipping cream, eggs, Splenda, and salt and cook for 10-12 minutes
2. Add butter, cabbage, toss to coat and mix well
3. Remove from heat add, walnuts and serve

Serves: **2**

Prep Time: **5** Minutes

Cook Time: **5** Minutes

Total Time: **10** Minutes

INGREDIENTS

- 2 tablespoons red wine vinegar
- 1 tablespoon water
- 1 tablespoon olive oil
- 1 tsp Dijon mustard
- ½ tsp garlic powder

DIRECTIONS

1. In a bowl mix all ingredients
2. Chill overnight and serve

Serves: *3*

Prep Time: *10*   Minutes

Cook Time: *50*   Minutes

Total Time: *60*   Minutes

INGREDIENTS

- 2 eggs
- 2 cups cottage cheese
- 1 red onion
- 1 pinch of pepper

DIRECTIONS

1. In a bowl mix all ingredients and pour into a casserole dish
2. Bake at 325 for 50 minutes
3. Remove and serve

Serves: **2**

Prep Time: **5**   Minutes

Cook Time: **5**   Minutes

Total Time: **10**   Minutes

INGREDIENTS

- ½ cup ketchup
- ¼ cup oil
- ¼ cup white vinegar
- 1 tsp lemon juice
- dash of pepper

DIRECTIONS

1. In a bowl mix all ingredients
2. Chill overnight and serve

Serves: *4*

Prep Time: *10*   Minutes

Cook Time: *10*   Minutes

Total Time: *20*   Minutes

INGREDIENTS

- ½ cup Kalamata olives
- 1 tsp capers
- ½ cup olive oil
- 1 tablespoon balsamic vinegar

DIRECTIONS

1. In a bowl chop olive and mix with crushed garlic
2. Add the rest of ingredients and mix well
3. Chill for 1-2 hours serve with asparagus or vegetables

Serves: **3**

Prep Time: **10**   Minutes

Cook Time: **10**   Minutes

Total Time: **20**   Minutes

INGREDIENTS

- 1 tablespoon oil
- 1 packet Portobello mushroom
- ½ cup maple syrup
- 1 tablespoon liquid smoke
- pinch of salt
- pinch of pepper

DIRECTIONS

1. In a bowl mix marinate the mushroom slices, mix with liquid smoke, maple syrup salt, and pepper
2. Cut the mushrooms into strips and marinade for 12-15 minutes
3. In a skillet cook mushrooms for 3-5 minutes or until browned
4. Remove, add lettuce, sliced tomato and serve

Serves: *4*

Prep Time: *10*   Minutes

Cook Time: *1*   Hour 30 Minutes

Total Time: *1*   Hour 30 Minutes

INGREDIENTS

- 2 lb. zucchini
- 1 onion
- ½ cup rice
- 1 can mushroom soup
- 2 beaten eggs
- 2 tablespoons butter
- 1 cup cheddar cheese

DIRECTIONS

1. Preheat the oven 325 F
2. In a bowl mix all ingredients
3. Pour mixture into a casserole dish
4. Top with grated cheese

Serves: **4**

Prep Time: **10**   Minutes

Cook Time: **30**   Minutes

Total Time: **40**   Minutes

INGREDIENTS

- 1 lb. noodles
- 1 cup parmesan cheese
- 2 cloves garlic
- 3 tablespoons coriander
- 5 tablespoons olive oil
- ¾ tsp salt
- ¼ tsp pepper

DIRECTIONS

1. Cook noodles according to directions and place in a bowl
2. Chop coriander and place in a bowl with crushed garlic
3. Mix with remaining ingredients, stir into the noodles
4. Serve when ready

Serves: *4*
Prep Time: *10*   Minutes

Cook Time: *2*   Hours 30 Minutes

Total Time: *2*   Hours 40 Hours

INGREDIENTS

- 3 chicken breasts
- ¼ cup olive oil
- ¼ cup balsamic vinegar
- 1 clove garlic

DIRECTIONS

1. In a bowl, add all ingredients
2. Add chicken and marinade for 3-4 hours
3. Grill and serve with vegetables

Serves: **4**
Prep Time: **10**   Minutes

Cook Time: **30**   Minutes

Total Time: **40**   Minutes

INGREDIENTS

- 3 salmon fillets
- ½ tsp dill weed
- ½ tsp parsley
- salt

DIRECTIONS

1. Season the salmon with pepper and parsley
2. Place each fillet on the grill at 325 F for 30 minutes
3. Remove and serve with vegetables

Serves: *4*

Prep Time: *10*   Minutes

Cook Time: *20*   Minutes

Total Time: *30*   Minutes

INGREDIENTS

- 1 red potato wedges
- 1 tablespoon rosemary
- 2 garlic cloves
- 1 tablespoon olive oil
- ¼ tsp onion powder
- ½ tsp salt
- ½ tsp pepper

DIRECTIONS

1. In a bowl mix potatoes and the rest of the ingredients
2. Toss to coat the potato wedges and place on a baking sheet
3. Bake for 20-25 minutes or until tender
4. Remove and serve

Serves: **1**

Prep Time: **10** Minutes

Cook Time: **10** Minutes

Total Time: **20** Minutes

INGREDIENTS

- 1 tsp olive oil
- 2 slices eggplant
- ½ tsp salt
- ½ tsp black pepper
- ½ cup goat cheese
- 2 sandwich rolls
- 2 slices tomato
- 1 cup arugula

DIRECTIONS

1. Preheat the oven to 275 F
2. In a skillet add eggplant, cook for 2-3 minutes per side, sprinkle with salt
3. Spread goat cheese and place rolls on a baking sheet
4. Bake at 250 F at 10-12 minutes, remove and serve

Serves: *4*

Prep Time: *20* Minutes

Cook Time: *1* Hour 20 Minutes

Total Time: *1* Hour 40 Minutes

INGREDIENTS

- 2 lemons
- 5 sage leaves
- 1 chicken
- 2 tsp olive oil
- ¾ lb. parsnips
- ¾ lb. carrots
- ½ lb. turnips
- 1 lb. fingerling potatoes
- 1 tablespoon thyme

DIRECTIONS

1. Preheat the oven to 400 F
2. Place sage and lemon slices under the skin of the chicken
3. Brush chicken with olive oil and place in roasting pan

4. Bake for at least 60 minutes at 325 F

5. Remove chicken to a plate

6. Roast vegetables for 40-45 minutes

7. Serve chicken with roasted vegetables

Serves: *4*

Prep Time: *10*   Minutes

Cook Time: *30*   Minutes

Total Time: *40*   Minutes

INGREDIENTS

- 2 lbs. sweet potatoes
- 1 tablespoon butter
- ½ unsweetened almond milk
- ½ tsp salt
- ½ tsp cinnamon
- ½ tsp ground ginger
- 1 pinch of nutmeg

DIRECTIONS

1. In a pot add sweet potatoes, water and bring to a boil for 12-15 minutes
2. Add remaining ingredients, cover cook until tender
3. Remove and serve

RASPBERRY TARTS

Serves: **4**

Prep Time: **10**   Minutes

Cook Time: **20**   Minutes

Total Time: **30**   Minutes

INGREDIENTS

- 1 package sugar cookie dough
- 1 package cream cheese
- ½ cup sugar
- zest of 1 orange
- ¼ tsp vanilla extract
- 30 raspberries

DIRECTIONS

1. Preheat the oven to 325 F
2. In a bowl place all ingredients and mix well, form small balls
3. Press each back into a greased tin and shape into a tin
4. Bake for 12-15 minutes, remove and set aside

5. In a bowl mix cream cheese, vanilla, orange zest, sugar and spoon cream cheese mixture into each tart

6. Serve when ready

Serves: **4**

Prep Time: **10**   Minutes

Cook Time: **20**   Minutes

Total Time: **30**   Minutes

INGREDIENTS

- 1 cup berries
- 1 tablespoon honey
- 1 tablespoon lemon juice
- 2 peaches
- 2 cups ice-cream

DIRECTIONS

1. In a blender add all ingredients and blend until smooth
2. Pour into a bowl and set aside
3. Place peach slices into the bowl, add ice cream, drizzle with berry sauce and serve

VANILLA BEAN PUDDING

Serves: *4*
Prep Time: *10*   Minutes

Cook Time: *20*   Minutes

Total Time: *30*   Minutes

INGREDIENTS

- 2 cups low-fat milk
- 1 vanilla bean
- ¾ cup sugar
- 3 tablespoons cornstarch
- ¼ tsp salt
- 3 tsp butter

- 2 egg yolks

DIRECTIONS

1. In a saucepan add milk, seeds, bean and bring to a boil
2. In another bowl mix cornstarch, salt, sugar, egg yolks and mix well
3. Stir egg yolk mixture into sugar mixture and cook for 8-10 minutes
4. Remove from heat add butter, remove vanilla bean and serve

TOMATO CROSTINI

Serves: **4**
Prep Time: **10**   Minutes

Cook Time: **20**   Minutes

Total Time: **30**   Minutes

INGREDIENTS

- ½ cup plum tomato
- 1 tablespoon basil
- 1 tablespoon green olives
- 1 tsp capers
- ¼ tsp balsamic vinegar
- ¼ tsp olive oil
- ¼ tsp salt
- dash of black pepper
- 1 garlic clove
- 4 slices bread baguette
- 1 garlic clove

DIRECTIONS

1. Preheat the oven to 350 F
2. Mix all ingredients except garlic clove and bread slices
3. Coat both sides of bread slices with cooking spray and arrange in a single layer on a baking sheet
4. Bake at 350 F for 5-6 minutes per side
5. Remove and rub 1 side with garlic and tomato mixture

Serves: *1*

Prep Time: *5*   Minutes

Cook Time: *5*   Minutes

Total Time: *10*   Minutes

INGREDIENTS

- 1 cup cornflakes
- 1 cup low-fat milk
- 1 cup berries

DIRECTIONS

1. In a bowl place all ingredients
2. Mix well and serve

Serves: *4*

Prep Time: *5*   Minutes

Cook Time: *5*   Minutes

Total Time: *10*   Minutes

INGREDIENTS

- 2 16 oz. cherries
- ½ cup honey
- 1 cup yogurt
- 1 tablespoon lemon juice
- salt

DIRECTIONS

1. In a bowl add all ingredients and blend until smooth
2. Pour into a bowl and serve

Serves: *12*
Prep Time: *10*   Minutes

Cook Time: *20*   Minutes

Total Time: *30*   Minutes

INGREDIENTS

- 1 cup coconut flour
- ½ cup coconut oil
- ¾ coconut milk
- 1 tsp vanilla extract
- zest of one lemon
- ½ cup maple syrup
- ½ tsp salt
- ¼ tsp baking powder
- ¼ tsp baking soda
- 1 egg

DIRECTIONS

1. Preheat the oven to 300 F
2. In a bowl mix coconut milk, egg, coconut oil, egg, lemon juice, extract, and maple syrup

3. In another bowl mix baking powder, baking soda, coconut flour and fold the milk mixture and mix well

4. Form 12-13 balls and bake for 15 minutes

5. Remove and serve

CHRISTMAS PUNCH

Serves: **12**

Prep Time: **5** Minutes

Cook Time: **5** Minutes

Total Time: **10** Minutes

INGREDIENTS

- 60 oz. cranberry juice
- 1 L diet coke
- 1 cup cranberries
- 1 lime
- 1 cup ice cubes

DIRECTIONS

1. Pour cranberry juice and diet coke in a bowl and add cranberries, limes and ice cubes

2. Serve when ready

Serves: *4*

Prep Time: *10* Minutes

Cook Time: *20* Minutes

Total Time: *30* Minutes

INGREDIENTS

- 2 can salmon
- 1 egg
- 1 tablespoon olive oil
- 1 onion
- ¼ potatoes
- salt

DIRECTIONS

1. Preheat the oven to 350 F
2. In a bowl mix all ingredients together and form patties
3. Bake for 15-20 minutes
4. Remove and serve

Serves: *4*

Prep Time: *10* Minutes

Cook Time: *30* Minutes

Total Time: *40* Minutes

INGREDIENTS

- 1 box cake mix
- 1 egg
- 1 can pumpkin
- 1 tsp cinnamon
- ¾ cup chocolate chips

DIRECTIONS

1. Preheat the oven to 325 F
2. Mix all ingredients and pour into a greased muffin pan
3. Bake for 18-20 minutes, remove and serve

Serves: *2*

Prep Time: *5*   Minutes

Cook Time: *5*   Minutes

Total Time: *10*   Minutes

INGREDIENTS

- 1 can chicken breast
- 1 stalk celery
- ½ cup mayonnaise
- 3 leaves romaine
- 1 oz. blue cheese
- 1 ripe tomato
- 1 cucumber

DIRECTIONS

1. In a bowl mix all ingredients and mix well
2. Serve with dressing

Serves: **2**

Prep Time: **5**   Minutes

Cook Time: **5**   Minutes

Total Time: **10**   Minutes

INGREDIENTS

- 1 lb. strip steak
- 5 cups romaine lettuce
- 1 cucumber
- 3 radishes
- 1/3 cup onion
- 1 cup tomatoes
- 1 ribs celery
- 1 cup broccoli florets

DIRECTIONS

1. In a bowl mix all ingredients and mix well
2. Serve with dressing

Serves: **2**

Prep Time: **5** Minutes

Cook Time: **5** Minutes

Total Time: **10** Minutes

INGREDIENTS

- 1 cup romaine lettuce
- 1 cup arugula
- 1 cucumber
- ½ cup red onion
- 2 oranges
- 2 tablespoons walnuts
- 2 tablespoons walnut oil
- 1 oz. blue cheese

DIRECTIONS

1. In a bowl mix all ingredients and mix well
2. Serve with dressing

Serves: **2**

Prep Time: **5**   Minutes

Cook Time: **5**   Minutes

Total Time: **10**   Minutes

INGREDIENTS

- 1 lb. red potatoes
- ¼ cup red onions
- ¼ lb. green beans
- ¼ cup tomato halves
- ¼ tsp rosemary
- 1 tsp olive oil

ROSEMARY VINAIGRETTE:

- 1 tablespoon olive oil
- 1 tablespoon red wine vinegar
- 1 tsp Dijon mustard
- ¼ tsp rosemary

DIRECTIONS

1. In a bowl mix all ingredients and mix well
2. Serve with dressing

Serves: **2**

Prep Time: **5** Minutes

Cook Time: **5** Minutes

Total Time: **10** Minutes

INGREDIENTS

- 1 tablespoon mayonnaise
- 1 tablespoon lemon juice
- 1 apple
- 1 cup red grapes
- ½ cup cranberries
- ½ cup walnuts
- 12 cup celery
- 6 lettuce leaves

DIRECTIONS

1. **In a bowl mix all ingredients and mix well**
2. **Serve with dressing**

Serves: **2**

Prep Time: **5**   Minutes

Cook Time: **5**   Minutes

Total Time: **10** Minutes

INGREDIENTS

- 1 tablespoon sherry vinegar
- 3 blood oranges
- 1 tsp Dijon mustard
- 1 tablespoon olive oil
- ½ tsp salt
- ½ tsp pepper
- 1 duck leg
- 5 cups salad greens
- ½ cup hazelnuts

DIRECTIONS

1. In a bowl mix all ingredients and mix well
2. Serve with dressing

Serves: *2*
Prep Time: *5*   Minutes

Cook Time: *5*   Minutes

Total Time: *10*   Minutes

INGREDIENTS

- 1 can peeled tomatoes
- 1 bunch cilantro
- 1 onion
- 1 garlic clove
- salt

DIRECTIONS

1. In a bowl mix all ingredients and mix well
2. Serve with dressing

Serves: **2**

Prep Time: **5**   Minutes

Cook Time: **5**   Minutes

Total Time: ***10*** Minutes

INGREDIENTS

- 1 can unsweetened pineapple
- 1 package cherry gelatin
- 1 tablespoon lemon juice
- ½ cup artificial sweetener
- 1 cup cranberries
- 1 orange
- 1 cup celery
- ½ cup pecans

DIRECTIONS

1. In a bowl mix all ingredients and mix well
2. Serve with dressing

Serves: **2**

Prep Time: **5**   Minutes

Cook Time: **5**   Minutes

Total Time: **10**   Minutes

INGREDIENTS

- 1 eggplant
- 1 onion
- 1 can black olives
- 1 jar Spanish olives
- ½ cup cider vinegar
- 1-quart tomato sauce

DIRECTIONS

1. In a bowl mix all ingredients and mix well
2. Serve with dressing

Serves: **2**

Prep Time: **5**   Minutes

Cook Time: **5**   Minutes

Total Time: **10** Minutes

INGREDIENTS

- 1 chicken breast
- Cajun spice
- 2 tablespoons hot sauce
- 1 cup romaine lettuce
- 1 tablespoon Caesar dressing
- 1 tablespoon parmesan cheese

DIRECTIONS

1. In a bowl mix all ingredients and mix well
2. Serve with dressing

CANTALOUPE SOUP

Serves: **4**

Prep Time: **10** Minutes

Cook Time: **30** Minutes

Total Time: **40** Minutes

INGREDIENTS

- 1 cantaloupe
- 1 tsp ginger
- ½ tsp nutmeg
- ¼ cup sour cream

DIRECTIONS

1. Cut cantaloupes in half, remove seeds and refrigerate
2. In a blender add sour cream, melon, spices and blend until smooth
3. Refrigerate for an hour, remove pour soup into bowls and serve

Serves: **4**

Prep Time: **10** Minutes

Cook Time: **30** Minutes

Total Time: **40** Minutes

INGREDIENTS

- 5 tablespoons olive oil
- 1 onion
- 1 clove garlic
- 1 potato
- ½ lb. pumpkin
- 2 carrots
- 1 celery stalk
- 1 broccoli head
- 1 zucchini
- 1 leek
- 8 cherry tomatoes
- 1 cup peas
- 1 L water
- 1 cube vegetable bouillon
- a handful of rice vermicelli

- ½ tsp salt
- few basil leaves

DIRECTIONS

1. In a pot add onion, garlic, vegetables and cook until soft
2. Add water, bouillon, peas and bring to a boil
3. Simmer for 12-15 minutes, add rice vermicelli, cook for 5-10 minutes
4. When ready remove and server with parmesan cheese

TOMATO PARMESAN SOUP

Serves: **4**

Prep Time: **10** Minutes

Cook Time: **35** Minutes

Total Time: **45** Minutes

INGREDIENTS

- 1 tablespoon olive oil

- 1 cup celery
- 1 cup carrots
- 1 cup onion
- 1 tablespoon dried basil
- 1 tsp dried oregano
- ¼ tsp bay leaf
- 26 oz. canned tomatoes
- 3 cups chicken broth
- ¼ cup butter
- ¼ cup four
- 1 cup parmesan
- 1 cup skim milk

DIRECTIONS

1. In a pot add onion, celery, carrots, bay leaf, tomatoes, basil, oregano, chicken broth and bring to a boil
2. Reduce heat and simmer for 18-20 minutes or until tender
3. In a skillet add butter, flour, 3 cup soup, and stir
4. Simmer until soup begins to thicken, stir in parmesan, skim milk, pepper and simmer for 15-18 minutes
5. Remove and serve

Serves: **4**

Prep Time: **10**   Minutes

Cook Time: **30**   Minutes

Total Time: **40**   Minutes

INGREDIENTS

- 2 tablespoons olive oil
- 2/3 cup spinach
- ¼ cup onion
- ½ cup red wine
- 1 tsp garlic
- 1 tablespoon basil
- 1 cup tomatoes
- 1 tsp oregano
- 1 cup tomatoes
- 1 oz. prosciutto
- 1 cup chicken broth

DIRECTIONS

1. **In a saucepan add garlic, onion, crushed tomatoes, broth, spinach, wine, herbs and bring to a boil**

2. Add ham, reduce heat and simmer for 30-35 minutes

3. When ready, remove from heat garnish with cheese and serve

STUFFED PEPPER SOUP

Serves: *4*

Prep Time: *10* Minutes

Cook Time: *35* Minutes

Total Time: *45* Minutes

INGREDIENTS

- 1 lb. ground beef
- 1 bell pepper
- 1 cup onion
- 1 can diced tomatoes
- 1 can tomato sauce
- 1 can chicken broth
- ½ tsp thyme
- ½ tsp dried sage

- 1 cup rice

DIRECTIONS

1. In a pot add beef, onions, peppers and cook until brown
2. Add tomato sauce, thyme, sage, tomatoes and simmer for 35-40 minutes
3. Add cooked rice and stir
4. When ready remove from heat, add cheese and serve

CREAMED CORN AND SPINACH STEW

Serves: *2*
Prep Time: *10* Minutes

Cook Time: *35* Minutes

Total Time: *45* Minutes

INGREDIENTS

- 2 cans tomato soup
- 3 cups water

- 2 cans creamed corn
- 2 cans corn kernel
- 2 cups spinach
- 2 cups tomato
- 2 tablespoons chili powder
- 1 can tomato paste
- salt

DIRECTIONS

1. In a pot add all ingredients and stir well
2. Cook on high heat for 15-18 minutes
3. Reduce heat on medium and simmer for another 15-18 minutes, stir well and serve

GINGER SOUP

Serves: *4*
Prep Time: *10* Minutes

Cook Time: *30* Minutes

Total Time: *40* Minutes

INGREDIENTS

- 2 tsp canola oil
- ¼ cup shallots
- 2 cups sweet potato
- 1 cup carrots
- 1 tablespoon ginger
- 1 tsp curry powder
- 2 cups chicken broth
- ¼ tsp salt

DIRECTIONS

1. In a saucepan add shallots and sauté for 4-5 minutes
2. Add the rest of ingredients and bring to a boil
3. Reduce heat and simmer for 25-30 minutes
4. Pour soup in a food processor and blend until smooth
5. When ready serve with salt and pepper

Serves: *3*

Prep Time: *10*   Minutes

Cook Time: *30*   Minutes

Total Time: *40*   Minutes

INGREDIENTS

- ½ tsp olive oil
- 1 onion
- ½ tsp garlic
- 1 carrot
- 1 cup vegetable stock
- 1 bay leaf
- ¼ cup lentils
- ¾ cup dried tomatoes
- ½ tsp thyme
- ½ tsp basil

DIRECTIONS

1. In a saucepan add onion, garlic, carrot and sauté for 5-6 minutes

2. Add water, stock, remaining ingredients and bring to a boil

3. Reduce heat and simmer for 18-20 minutes

4. Remove bay leaf and serve

SAVORY MOROCCAN

Serves: **4**

Prep Time: **10** Minutes

Cook Time: **20** Minutes

Total Time: **30** Minutes

INGREDIENTS

- 3 cups vegetable stock
- 1 can diced tomatoes
- 1 cup zucchini
- ½ cup canned chickpeas
- 3 artichoke hearts
- ¼ cup whole-wheat couscous
- ½ cup parsley

- ½ cup raisins
- 1 scallion
- ½ tsp cinnamon
- ½ tsp cayenne
- ¼ tsp basil
- ¼ tsp oregano

DIRECTIONS

1. In a pot add water, stock, and remaining ingredients
2. Bring to a boil and simmer for 8-10 minutes
3. Add salt, pepper and serve

CHICKEN & BROWN RICE

Serves: *4*

Prep Time: *10*   Minutes

Cook Time: *40*   Minutes

Total Time: *50*   Minutes

INGREDIENTS

- 1 tsp olive oil
- 1 lb. chicken breast
- 1 carrot
- 1 celery stalk
- ½ leek
- ½ cup brown rice
- 1 tsp thyme
- 1 can diced tomatoes

DIRECTIONS

1. In a saucepan add chicken and sauté until cooked
2. Transfer to a plate and set aside
3. In the saucepan add celery, leek, carrot, rice, thyme and sauté for 4-5 minutes
4. Chop chicken and add back to saucepan
5. Add stock, tomatoes and simmer for 30 minutes on low heat
6. Remove from heat, add pepper and serve

Serves: *1*
Prep Time: *5* Minutes

Cook Time: *5* Minutes

Total Time: *10* Minutes

INGREDIENTS

- 6 oz. water
- 1 cup pineapple
- 1 orange
- 1 carrot
- 1 tablespoon chia seeds
- ½ tsp ginger
- 1 handful baby spinach

DIRECTIONS

1. In a blender place all ingredients and blend until smooth
2. Pour smoothie in a glass and serve

Serves: *1*

Prep Time: *5*   Minutes

Cook Time: *5*   Minutes

Total Time: *10*   Minutes

INGREDIENTS

- 4 oz. water
- 1 mango
- 1 kiwifruit
- 1 cup kale

DIRECTIONS

1. In a blender place all ingredients and blend until smooth
2. Pour smoothie in a glass and serve

Serves: *1*

Prep Time: *5*   Minutes

Cook Time: *5*   Minutes

Total Time: *10*   Minutes

INGREDIENTS

- 5 oz. water
- 1 banana
- 3 strawberries
- 1 orange
- 1 baby spinach

DIRECTIONS

1. **In a blender place all ingredients and blend until smooth**
2. **Pour smoothie in a glass and serve**

Serves: **1**

Prep Time: **5** Minutes

Cook Time: **5** Minutes

Total Time: **10** Minutes

INGREDIENTS

- 5 oz. water
- 1 cup cantaloupe
- 1 mango
- 3 strawberries
- 1 handful baby spinach

DIRECTIONS

1. In a blender place all ingredients and blend until smooth
2. Pour smoothie in a glass and serve

Serves: *1*

Prep Time: *5*   Minutes

Cook Time: *5*   Minutes

Total Time: *10*   Minutes

INGREDIENTS

- 5 oz. water
- 1 banana
- ¼ red grapefruit
- ¼ cup pineapple
- ¼ cup cucumber
- ¼ cup parsley

DIRECTIONS

1. In a blender place all ingredients and blend until smooth
2. Pour smoothie in a glass and serve

Serves: *1*
Prep Time: **5**   Minutes

Cook Time: **5**   Minutes

Total Time: *10*   Minutes

INGREDIENTS

- 1 cup cherries
- 1 cup strawberries
- 1 banana
- 1 cup almond milk

DIRECTIONS

1. In a blender place all ingredients and blend until smooth
2. Pour smoothie in a glass and serve

Serves: *1*

Prep Time: *5* Minutes

Cook Time: *5* Minutes

Total Time: *10* Minutes

INGREDIENTS

- 1 cup frozen berries
- ½ cup blueberries
- 1 tablespoon soy protein
- 1 cup spinach
- 1 cup yogurt

DIRECTIONS

1. In a blender place all ingredients and blend until smooth
2. Pour smoothie in a glass and serve

Serves: **1**

Prep Time: **5** Minutes

Cook Time: **5** Minutes

Total Time: **10** Minutes

INGREDIENTS

- 1 white tea bag
- 2/3 cup water
- 1 wedge lime juice
- 1 cup ice cubes

DIRECTIONS

1. In a blender place all ingredients and blend until smooth
2. Pour smoothie in a glass and serve

Serves: *1*

Prep Time: *5*   Minutes

Cook Time: *5*   Minutes

Total Time: *10*   Minutes

INGREDIENTS

- ~   1 banana
- ~   1 yogurt
- ~   ½ cup non-fat milk

DIRECTIONS

1. In a blender place all ingredients and blend until smooth
2. Pour smoothie in a glass and serve

Serves: *1*

Prep Time: *5* Minutes

Cook Time: *5* Minutes

Total Time: *10* Minutes

INGREDIENTS

- 1 banana
- 3 tablespoons peanut butter
- 1 cup rice milk
- 1 tablespoon flax seeds

DIRECTIONS

1. In a blender place all ingredients and blend until smooth
2. Pour smoothie in a glass and serve

Printed in Great Britain
by Amazon

62329348R00061